Low Carb - 21 Day Diet Plan

The Most Effective Formula For Rapid Weight Loss

Table of Content

Introduction

Thank you for purchasing this book "**Low Carb - 21 Day Diet Plan**".

Do you want to lead a healthier life, lose weight or reverse type-2 diabetes? However varied your reason might be for choosing a low carb diet, you will definitely be able to reap all the benefits that a low carb diet has to offer if you follow the diet strictly. In this book, you will learn everything that you need to know about a low carb diet.

The topics that are covered in this book include the basics of what a low carb diet is, the health benefits of following a low carb diet, the common mistakes that people tend to make while following the low carb diet and how you can avoid them, the different mental strategies that will help you in sticking to your diet, different benefits of one skillet cooking, the list of foods that you should eat and avoid, a 21 day meal plan and a plethora of low carb recipes for all meals – from breakfast to dinner, and for all courses from appetizer, main course, to desserts and smoothies!

As the name of this book suggests, this book focuses on the consumption of limited amounts of foods that are rich in starch and sugar like bread, rice, pasta, desserts, fruits and even a couple of vegetables. A diet that is based on consumption of low carbohydrates focuses on the consumption of foods that are rich in proteins and certain natural fats. This book will help in explaining how you can manage to eat as much as you want while you are decreasing your level of blood sugar, cholesterol and also lose weight without having to starve yourself.

Equipped with the information given in this book, you can definitely lead a healthier life, full of delicious, healthy and nutritious foods. You will need to follow the diet strictly; a little bit of extra commitment surely goes a long way.

Thank you for purchasing this book and I hope you enjoy the recipes that have been provided in this book.

Chapter 1: What is a Low-Carb Diet?

The evolution of human beings took over a million years. From our hunter-gatherer ancestors, we have come a long way. Our ancestors not only survived, they thrived without consuming large amounts of carbohydrates on daily basis. They ate whatever food they could gather from the environment. They didn't have any processed food like bread, pasta or even any starchy foods like rice and potatoes. The consumption of starchy foods started only after the development of agriculture, a few thousand years ago.

The industrial revolution started 100 to 200 years ago and this lead to factories that are capable of manufacturing large quantities of pure sugar and refined flour. But our bodies didn't have sufficient time to get genetically adapted to all these processed foods. During the80s, the western world was gripped by the fear of becoming "fat". So called low-fat products kept popping up all over the place. But consuming less of the dietary fat that your body needs, you will end up consuming more carbohydrates to satisfy your hunger. It's around the same time that our world was plagued by the onslaught of obesity and diabetes. The USA, the most fat-phobic country, was hit the hardest.

The carbohydrates that we consume are broken down into simple sugars during digestion. These sugars are then absorbed into the blood and this in turn results in the rise of the glucose levels in blood. When there's an increase in the glucose level, the production of a fat storing hormone, insulin increases as well. Pancreas is responsible for the production of insulin. When produced in large amounts, it obstructs the burning of fat and stores all the surplus nutrients within the fat cells.

This leads to an apparent shortage of nutrients in the blood after a while and creates hunger pangs and cravings for something sweet. Usually this is the point where a person would eat again. This starts the process all over again and this vicious cycle leads to weight gain.

On the other hand, when you decrease your intake of carbohydrates, the glucose level in the blood is more stable and lower quantities of insulin are released by pancreas. This increases the burning of fat within the cells. This leads to fat loss, especially in areas around the abdomen in obese individuals.

A low carbohydrate diet facilitates the easier usage of fat reserves because the release of fat is no longer obstructed by high levels of insulin. This is the reason why the consumption of fatty foods makes you feel fuller for longer than when you eat carbs. According to studies that have been conducted regarding the effects of a low-carb diet, it's been observed that when people tend to eat all that they want to when on a low-carb diet their caloric intake tends to drop considerably. So, you needn't count calories or weigh your food while on a low-carb diet. If you don't believe me, why don't you try it out for a few weeks to see the difference for yourself?

None of the animals in nature need any additional assistance or any nutritional expertise or a calories chart for their meals. As long as they eat the food that their bodies are designed to eat, they maintain their normal weight and remain disease free. Then why would human beings be an exception? Various scientific studies show that people tend to not only shed weight but can also manage their blood pressure, blood sugar and cholesterol levels while on a low-carb diet.

If you don't eat starch and sugar right away, you might experience certain side effects. These side effects are temporary and are caused when your body is getting adjusted to the low-carb diet. These side effects would be mild and last for a few days. The most common side effects are headaches, fatigue, dizziness and irritability. Once your body gets acclimatized to burning fat for generating energy, these side effects would fade away. Drinking lots of water and slightly increasing your salt intake will minimize these symptoms.

Chapter 2: Why Chose a Low-carb Diet?

Reduction in Appetite

One of the worst side effects of dieting is hunger. This is also one of the main reasons why many tend to give op on their diets. One of the best things about a low-carb diet is that it leads to an automatic reduction in one's appetite. When you tend to cut down on carbs and instead consume more protein and fat, not only will you be consuming lesser calories but you will also feel fuller and end up eating considerably smaller portions. This means that you will end up eating fewer calories without even trying to do so.

Leads to Effective Weight Loss

The simplest and effective ways to lose weight is by cutting down on carbs. Even when you don't actively restrict your calorie consumption, you tend to shed weight easily. A low-carb diet helps in getting rid of all excess water from the body. Kidneys tend to get rid of the excess sodium because of low levels of insulin and this leads to rapid weight loss during the first two weeks of the diet. You can lose weight without having to starve yourself. It is better to think of eating low-carb foods as a lifestyle and not just a diet if you really want to maintain your weight.

Fat Loss is Usually from the Abdominal Cavity

Not all the fat that's present in your body is the same. Depending upon the location of where this fat is store, it would have an effect on your health. We tend to have subcutaneous fat or fat that's present under the skin and visceral fat or fat in the abdominal cavity. Visceral fat tends to get lodged around the different organs. Having a lot of fat in this region can lead to a spike in insulin levels, inflammation and even metabolic dysfunction. Low-carb diets have proven to be successful in eliminating abdominal fat. Over a period of time, this will lead to reducing the risk of heart diseases and diabetes.

Reduction in the Level of triglycerides

Triglycerides are fat molecules and they are a risk factor for heart diseases. Consumption of carbohydrates, especially simple sugars like fructose, elevates the level of triglycerides in the body. When the amount of carbs that you consume has been reduced then this leads to a reduction in the level of triglycerides as well.

Increase in the Levels of Good Cholesterol

HDL or High Density Lipoprotein is referred to as good cholesterol. Technically these can't be called as cholesterol and they are lipoproteins that are responsible for carrying cholesterol in the blood. LDL is responsible for carrying cholesterol from the liver and transport it to the rest of the body and HDL is responsible for shipping the cholesterol from the rest of the body to the liver, where it can either be reused or removed from the body. The higher the level of HDL is the lower is your risk for heart diseases and one of the best ways in which you can do this is by consuming foods that have natural dietary fats. Therefore, it doesn't come, as a surprise that your HDL level would improve when on a low-carb diet.

Reduced Levels of Blood Sugar and Insulin

The carbohydrates that you eat are broken down into sugars during digestion. Then these sugars enter the blood stream and this increases the level of blood sugars. When the blood sugar level rises, the body releases a hormone called insulin and this transports glucose to cells for either being burnt for energy or stored. For a healthy individual, a spike in sugar level is neutralized by insulin, but for those who suffer from problems with this system their body develops insulin resistance. Insulin resistance is the condition where the cells fail to recognize insulin and this makes it extremely difficult for the body to move blood sugar into the cells. This causes type-2 diabetes, where the body can't produce sufficient insulin to reduce the blood sugar level. The simple answer to fighting this problem is by cutting carbs. If you remove the need for all the additional insulin, the excess blood sugar also goes away with it.

Reduction in the Level of Blood Pressure

Hypertension or elevated level of blood pressure is a risk factor for a host of diseases targeting the heart, kidneys and other major organs. A low-carb diet helps in reducing the blood pressure and this in turn reduces the risk of other diseases as well.

Effective in Combating Metabolic Syndrome

Metabolic syndrome is a condition that's associated with diabetes and various heart diseases. The usually symptoms are obesity, high blood pressure, high blood sugar, high triglycerides and low level of HDL. All the five symptoms can be reduced considerably by following a low-carb diet. By following this diet and not slipping into your old eating habits, metabolic syndrome can be controlled.

Improves LDL Cholesterol

LDL refers to Low Density Lipoprotein and this is usually referred to as bad cholesterol. But this isn't cholesterol and it is in fact a lipoprotein that is responsible for carrying cholesterol from the liver to the rest of the body. People with elevated levels of LDL are more prone to heart attacks. A low-carb diet will help in turning the small LDL particles in the blood stream into larger particles and also reduces the number of LDL molecules in the bloodstream. Small LDL particles are responsible for increasing the risk of heart diseases.

Considered to be Therapeutic for Various Brain Disorders

Glucose is extremely important for the proper functioning of the brain. Some parts of the brain are capable of only burning glucose. This is the reason why the liver produces glucose by breaking down proteins if you don't consume carbs. A major portion of the brain is capable of burning ketones that are formed when the carb intake is low. This is the mechanism that operates in any low-carb diet like the Ketogenic diet that has been used in treating epilepsy in children who haven't been responding to drugs or other lines of treatment. In most of the cases of epilepsy, a low-carb diet has been helpful in reducing the symptoms for a great extent and now it is being considered to help in managing other disorders like Alzheimer's and Parkinson's.

Chapter 3: Mental Strategies to Help Lose Weight

It is very important that you keep yourself motivated while you are trying to lose weight. At times it might get really difficult to stay on track and focus on your diet, or you might just feel like quitting. In order to avoid these things, here are a few mental strategies that will help you stay focused.

Visualization

If you really want to let go of your old habits, then you will need to see yourself in a positive light. If you want to lose weight, then picture your future self. Visualize how you would want to look six months or perhaps a year down the line and think about how good you would feel without those extra kilos weighing you down. Put up pictures of yourself when you were thinner, to serve as a reminder of what you are working for. Do you want to wear the latest bikini that you have been crushing on? Well, every time you feel discouraged all that you need to do is just visualize yourself in that bikini!

Keep Your Expectations Realistic

Your expectations need to be realistic and attainable. If you have unrealistic expectations then you are just setting yourself up for failure. Ask yourself simple questions, how much weight would you want to lose in the next 12 months? Is it 12 or 24 pounds? That's about one or two pounds a month and it's perfectly doable.

You can reevaluate your weight goals after every 6 months. But you will need to make sure that your expectations are manageable.

Setting Small Goals

You should make a list of smaller goals that will help you in achieving your actual weight loss goal. These small goals could relate to things that you would like to change about your lifestyle without turning your life upside down. These small goals will ultimately help you in achieving your main goal. Examples of small goals could be promising you to eat more vegetables every day, working out for about 30 minutes every day or abstaining from alcohol or junk food for a month! Your small goal could be anything. It could perhaps be something as simple as waking up early in the morning and going for a walk or a jog. Change can be difficult. Instead of trying to change everything at once, it would be more effective if you make small changes and do so gradually, instead of rushing into it.

Support System

You will need a support system to keep you going when times get tough. Your friends and family members could be your support system. Explain to them why the diet means a lot and how you would want to achieve your weight goals. If you ever feel like quitting, then your support system will provide you the motivation to keep going.

Plan of action

Planning is very important. Make it a point to plan for the next day before going to bed. Planning ahead will help you prepare yourself mentally for getting through the day. When you know ahead what you are supposed to do, it becomes easier to go through the day and the chances of slipping back into your old eating habits would reduce too. Your health should be your priority and you should take such steps that will help you in cultivating healthier habits to achieve your goal.

Rewards Yourself

Reward yourself whenever you do something that will put you a step closer to your goal. If you have managed to follow the diet for a week or have managed to fight your craving for your favorite slice of pastry, you should reward yourself. You can treat yourself to a manicure or does anything that would make you feel good. Every time you achieve one of the mini goals that you have set for yourself, remember to reward yourself. This will keep you motivated to achieve your goal.

Ditching Your Old Habits

If you really want to lose weight, then you can't continue doing things the way you used to. You will need to overcome your old habits. It will take a while to overcome but you can eventually overcome them. You will have to identify the areas or activities that you might be engaging in that are leading to weight gain and then turn them around, one-by-one. For instance, if you like watching TV in the evening, then you can start out by switching your evening snack from chips to a piece of fruit. Then you can switch to a calorie free drink and then perhaps you can start exercising while watching TV. Another way to get rid of your old habits would be by simply getting rid of all of the unhealthy foodstuff from your home.

Keep Track

You will need to keep a journal to track your progress. Include information about what you eat, the amount of time spent on exercise, your emotions and also your weight and weekly measurements. This will help in reinforcing positive thoughts and behavior. Maintaining a journal will make you feel accountable and responsible to your own self.

Chapter 4: Benefits of One-Skillet Cooking

You might think that the "frying" pan is perhaps bad for you. After all, you make use of it for cooking your burgers and frying up bacon rashers. According to nutritionists as well as chefs, a skillet is a very versatile cooking tool and it can be used for a cooking a healthy and delicious meal. Well, in today's world everyone is busy and no one really has got the time to cook at home. A one-pan meal can be really easy to cook and extremely healthy when compared to the unhealthy alternative of perhaps microwaving a frozen dinner or eating takeout.

The concept of a one-pan meal not only ensures that the clutter caused due to cooking is minimal but it's extremely easy as well. Cooking in a skillet usually means that you will first cook the protein, then cook the vegetables in it, toss everything back in along with any sauce, wine or broth to act as flavoring agents and for enhancing the flavors as well. Ten or fifteen minutes later, dinner is ready to be served. Not only is it as simple as that, but it will definitely taste better than frozen meals. All the flavors and nutrients from all the components in the meal have been sealed in one skillet and you haven't lost any flavor.

One of the best features of a one-skillet meal is that the recipes generally include vegetables, protein as well as a little bit of carbohydrates (if required). All this is simply cooked together. Combining all the ingredients in the same skillet means that all the flavors would be sealed and blended together. The textures of individual elements would be sealed and their individual flavors would be retained as well.

Another advantage is that you can make use of cheaper and tougher cuts of meat and just let them simmer for longer to make a hearty soup or stew.

This also helps in creating sauces from the natural juices secreted by the various ingredients. If you don't have the time to cook, you will simply need to chuck all the ingredients into the skillet and just let it cook slowly. It is definitely simpler to reheat things without having to change the container.

Chapter 5: The Most Common Mistakes

In this chapter, let's take a look at some of the most common mistakes that people tend to make when on a low-carb diet.

Getting the Basics Wrong

You don't really need to take a specific course to understand what a low-carb diet is all about. It simply means restricting the amount of carbs that you are consuming. But this doesn't mean that you should simply be eating meat all day long. You need to get your basics about low-carb eating right. You will need to have knowledge about the kind of foods that you can and cannot eat.

Giving Up Easily

There are various approaches to a low-carb diet and you might end up making a few mistakes along the way. You needn't worry about it. It might take longer for results to show on you than it did for someone else. But this doesn't mean that you should quit. Tweak the diet a little to suit your needs and don't give up easily. Stick to the diet for at least a month to see positive results.

Not Eating Sufficient Vegetables

Vegetables are not only a source of nutrients and carbs for you, but they provide essential dietary fiber that helps in better absorption and digestion of food. Skipping vegetables altogether or not eating the required amount of vegetables is a wrong thing to do. You need to eat at least 5 to 6 servings of non-starchy vegetables every day.

Not Enough Fats

This can really be problematic. All fats aren't bad and you shouldn't avoid them completely. Certain dietary fats are essential to help in the better absorption of nutrients in the body. Consuming low fat or diet foods are a very bad idea; in fact these products are harmful because of all the processed ingredients that they make use of. Fatty foods won't slow down your progress. In fact eating less of fatty protein while on a low-carb diet will simply give you hunger pangs. Nothing ruins a diet like hunger does.

No Enough Fiber

Vegetables and fruits are some sources of fiber that your body needs. You will need to educate yourself about all the different sources of fiber that are available and you can opt for the sources with the least amount of carbs in them.

Eating Too Much

It is true that you needn't count calories when you are on a low-carb diet. But this doesn't mean that calories don't count, at all! A low-carb diet is effective in helping cut down weight because it helps in controlling your appetite without trying to do so. Eating more of protein tends to satiate your hunger without adding too many calories when compared to a diet that's rich in carbohydrates. Let your appetite guide you. Eat only when you are hungry!

Lack of Planning

If you want to stick to the diet, then you will need to plan your meals well in advance. You will have to buy all the necessary ingredients and stock up your pantry. This will make sure that you don't slip back into your old eating habits. Whenever you have the time, you can cook batches of food and simply freeze it. You can heat up these meals whenever you want to. Planning your meals properly also means that you won't go hungry and give into your urge to snack on carbs.

Not Reading the Labels

It would be wise to stay away from processed food. Anything that looks like it was produced in a factory should be avoided. Whatever food item you are buying, you should check the list of ingredients that has been given. If you don't recognize any of the ingredients or see any hydrogenated fats or unsaturated fats mentioned on it, then you should avoid it. Not all foodstuffs that are supposed to be "low-carb" are actually low carb. So, you need to be careful while you are shopping for groceries.

Carb Creep

Everything might be going perfectly fine. You are probably losing those extra kilos and you are healthier. You get the urge to treat yourself to that piece of chocolate that you have been denying yourself or perhaps you want to start adding sugar to your daily cup of coffee. Carbs will start creeping back into your diet unless you are extremely careful about it. You can slowly add a few starchy foods but this doesn't mean that you start eating all carbohydrate rich foods.

The points mentioned above will definitely come in handy when you are following a low-carb diet and you will be able to successfully avoid some of the most common mistakes that people tend to make. You can always combine this diet with exercising for obtaining optimum results.

Chapter 6: Foods to Eat and Foods to Avoid

Now that you know the various advantages of following a low-carb diet and the way it works. You might be wondering about what you can and cannot eat while on this diet? This chapter will precisely help you this question.

There are certain things that you can eat and certain things that you should avoid at any cost. If you know this list, it will be easier for you to collect all the necessary groceries and when you have a fully stocked pantry with all the essential items, you won't slip back into your old ways of eating. You can eat meat, fish, eggs, vegetables, fruits, nuts, seeds, dairy products, fats and healthy oils. You cannot eat sugar, processed foods, wheat, rice, or any other diet foods. Let's look at an elaborate list of items that you can and cannot include while on a low-carb diet.

Foods to Avoid

Avoid all the seven foods that have been listed below, avoid them at any cost.

- Sugar: soft drinks, pre-packaged fruit drinks, sodas, agave, chocolates, candy, ice creams and anything else that has got processed sugar in it.
- Gluten: grains that have gluten like wheat, barley, rye and anything that has gluten. This means that you can't eat bread or pastas either.

- Trans-fat: anything that says, "trans-fat", "hydrogenated oils" or "partially hydrogenated oils" should be avoided like the plague.

- Omega-6 and vegetable oils: Soybean oil, sunflower oil, corn or canola oils and any other refined oils should be avoided.

- Artificial sweeteners: sucralose, saccharin, aspartame and other artificial sweeteners. These are as bad as or worse than sugar. You can instead make use of stevia.

- Diet or low-fat foods: there's nothing "diet" about all the so-called diet food available these days. Stay away from any food item that says "diet" or "low-fat".

- Processed foods: HPL or Highly Processed Foods should be avoided. Read the ingredients or the contents mentioned on the boxes even if it says "healthy". Anything that seems processed is probably processed, so stay away from it.

Foods to Eat

Your diet should be based on real, unprocessed foods that have low-carb content.

- Meat: beef, lamb, pork, chicken, turkey and other poultry meats. Grass-fed or organic meat is preferably.

- Fish: salmon, trout, haddock and any other fish is perfectly fine. The natural oils in fish are good for you.

- Eggs are the best source of Omega-3 fatty oils.

- Vegetables like spinach, broccoli, asparagus, cauliflower, squash, zucchini, carrots, cabbage and many more. It's best to avoid extremely starchy vegetables like potatoes during the first few weeks.
- Fruits: Apples, oranges, watermelon, muskmelon, blueberries, raspberries, strawberries, blackberries, cherries and other berries, that are rich in antioxidants.
- Nuts and seeds like almonds, walnuts, sunflower seeds, pumpkin seeds and so on.
- High-fat and full cream dairy products like milk, cheese, cream and yogurt.
- Fats and oils: extra virgin olive oil, coconut oil, lard, cod liver oil and sesame oil as well.

If you want to lose weight then go easy on cheese and nuts and restrict the amount of fruits that you consume as well.

Can Probably Eat

You can eat these foods only if you are active, exercise regularly and don't need to lose weight. You can afford to eat a few carbs every day, but in moderation.

- Tubers like potatoes, sweet potatoes and so on.
- Non-gluten grains like rice, oats and even quinoa.
- Legumes like lentils, black beans and other beans.
- Dark chocolate with cocoa content of above 70%.
- Dry wines without any added sugars or carbs.

Remember you can eat the above mentioned food items in

moderation and don't eat any of them if you don't want to slow down your progress. You can drink as much water and green tea as you want. Coffee without any sugar and you can have sugar-free carbonated drinks like sparkling water.

Chapter 7: 21 Day Meal Plan

Day 1
Breakfast - Stir Fry Eggs & Vegetables

Lunch - Ground Beef with Sliced Bell Peppers

Dinner - Crispy Carnitas, Three Minute Chocolate Cake

Snacks – handful of unsalted nuts like almonds or pecans

Day 2
Breakfast - Sausage & Egg Breakfast Bites

Lunch - Delicious Chili Cheese Dogs

Dinner - Bacon Wrapped Mini Meatloaves, Chocolate "Peanut Butter" Ice Cream with Chocolate Shell

Snacks – ½ cup plain, full fat Greek yogurt topped with fruit of your choice

Day 3
Breakfast - Cowboy Breakfast Skillet

Lunch - Low Carb Lettuce Wraps

Dinner - Pizza Topping Casserole, Magically Moist Almond Cake

Snacks – 1 bowl unsalted, un-buttered popcorn

Day 4
Breakfast - Broccoli & Cheese Mini Egg Omelets

Lunch - Carolina Style Barbeque Meatballs

Dinner - Swedish Meatballs, Sweet & Salty Fudge Bombs

Snacks – Carrot sticks with a gluten free hummus

Day 5

Breakfast - Tex-Mex Scramble

Lunch - Honey Mustard Cuban Pork Burgers

Dinner - Swedish Meatballs, Simple Blueberry Lemon Birthday Cake

Snacks – ½ cup Apple slices with a little string cheese

Day 6

Breakfast - Savory Cheese Chive Waffles

Lunch - Bora Bora Fireballs, Mexican Chocolate Coffee Cake

Dinner - Simple Herb Crusted Salmon, Salted Caramel Custard

Snacks – Ripe avocado mash spread on 2 rye crisps

Day 7

Breakfast - Cinnamon Roll Smoothie, with a handful of nuts

Lunch - Buttery Catfish in A Creamy Shallot Sauce, Simply Delicious Sugar Free Cheesecake

Dinner - Asian Inspired Chicken Wings, Healthy Strawberry Frozen Yogurt

Snacks – cucumber sticks with plain Greek yogurt

Day 8

Breakfast - Blueberry Oatmeal Smoothie with a hard-boiled egg

Lunch - Quick & Easy Low Carb Fish Sticks

Dinner - Delicious Chili Cheese Dogs, Dairy Free Dark Chocolate Mousse

Snacks – ½ cup cottage cheese with ½ cup fruit of your choice

Day 9

Breakfast - Broccoli & Cheese Mini Egg Omelets

Lunch - Bacon Wrapped Mini Meatloaves

Dinner - Asian Inspired Chicken Wings, Almond Coconut Bars

Snacks – celery sticks with some low carb peanut butter

Day 10

Breakfast - Blueberry & Spinach Smoothie, with a hard-boiled egg

Lunch - Crispy Carnitas

Dinner - Carolina Style Barbeque Meatballs, Salted Caramel
Custard

Snacks – Hardboiled egg with a sprinkling of cayenne or hot sauce

Day 11

Breakfast - Stir Fry Eggs & Vegetables

Lunch - Cheese Enchiladas

Dinner - Simple Herb Crusted Salmon, Simple Blueberry Lemon
Birthday Cake

Snacks - handful of unsalted mixed nuts, such as peanut, almond,
cashew nuts

Day 12

Breakfast - Purple Detox Smoothie with a handful of assorted nuts

Lunch - Asian Inspired Chicken Wings

Dinner - Crispy Carnitas, Healthy Strawberry Frozen Yogurt

Snacks –Un-buttered popcorn, topped with some cayenne and salt

Day 13

Breakfast - Blackberry Banana Bliss Smoothie with a hardboiled egg

Lunch - Pizza Topping Casserole

Dinner - Buttery Catfish in a Creamy Shallot Sauce, Magically Moist Almond Cake

Snacks – plain low fat Greek yogurt with apple slices

Day 14

Breakfast - Tex-Mex Scramble

Lunch - Cheese Enchiladas

Dinner - Ground Beef with Sliced Bell Peppers, Mexican Chocolate Coffee Cake

Snacks – Avocado mash on 2 rye crisps

Day 15

Breakfast- Blueberry & Spinach Smoothie, with a handful of assorted nuts

Lunch - Low Carb Lettuce Wraps

Dinner - Delicious Chili Cheese Dogs, Three Minute Chocolate Cake

Snacks - Carrot and celery sticks with a low carb condiment of your choice

Day 16

Breakfast - Blackberry Banana Bliss Smoothie with a handful of assorted nuts

Lunch - Swedish Meatballs

Dinner - Pizza Topping Casserole, Dairy Free Dark Chocolate

Mousse

Snacks – ½ cup low fat plain Greek yogurt with ½ cup fruits of your choice

Day 17
Breakfast - Sausage & Egg Breakfast Bites

Lunch - Bora Bora Fireballs

Dinner - Ground Beef with Sliced Bell Peppers, Simply Delicious Sugar Free Cheesecake

Snacks - celery sticks with some low carb peanut butter

Day 18
Breakfast - Savory Cheese Chive Waffles

Lunch - Cheesy Tuna Casserole

Dinner - Bacon Wrapped Mini Meatloaves, Sweet & Salty Fudge Bombs

Snacks - ½ cup Apple slices with a little string cheese

Day 19
Breakfast - Purple Detox Smoothie with a hard-boiled egg

Lunch - Buttery Catfish in a Creamy Shallot Sauce

Dinner - Honey Mustard Cuban Pork Burgers, Almond Coconut Bars

Snacks - ½ cup cottage cheese with ½ cup fruit of your choice

Day 20
Breakfast - Cowboy Breakfast Skillet

Lunch - Ground Beef with Sliced Bell Peppers

Dinner - Bora Bora Fireballs, Sweet & Salty Fudge Bombs

Snacks – handful of assorted nuts with ½ cup of plain Greek yogurt

Day 21

Breakfast - Cinnamon Roll Smoothie with a hardboiled egg

Lunch - Low Carb Lettuce Wraps

Dinner - Cheese Enchiladas, Chocolate "Peanut Butter" Ice Cream with Chocolate Shell

Snacks – Hardboiled egg with a sprinkling of cayenne or hot sauce

Chapter 8: Breakfast Recipes with Low Carb

Stir Fry Eggs & Vegetables

Ingredients:

- 2 tablespoon Coconut oil
- 4 eggs
- ½ cup spinach, finely chopped
- ½ cup Frozen Vegetable Mix (green beans, cauliflower, carrots, broccoli), thawed
- Cayenne powder, to taste
- Salt, to taste
- Pepper, to taste

Instructions:

1. Pour the coconut oil into a frying pan and heat over a medium high flame until lightly smoking.
2. Add the thawed mixed vegetables into the pan and heat for a few minutes.
3. Pour in the eggs and lightly scramble using a wooden spoon.
4. Add the salt, pepper and cayenne into the pan and mix well.
5. Add the chopped spinach to the pan and stir fry until cooked through. Serve hot and enjoy!

Sausage & Egg Breakfast Bites

Ingredients:

- 1 tablespoon olive oil + some for greasing
- 1/4 cup dark leafy greens, such as Swiss chard, kale, spinach, beet greens
- 5 eggs
- 1 cup uncooked sausage, crumbled
- Parsley, thyme, oregano or any other fresh herb to taste.

Instructions:

1. Crank up your oven to 375 degrees F and allow the oven to preheat.
2. Remove the stems from the greens and cut into strips.
3. Pour the olive oil into a pan and add the greens to the pan and toss well for a few minutes.
4. Add the crumbled sausage into the pan and heat until the sausage is cooked through.
5. Take the pan off the flame.
6. Whisk the eggs with a wire whisk and add the cooked sausage and greens to the eggs.
7. Grease an 8 x 8 inch pan with some oil.
8. Pour the eggs; veggie and sausage mix into the pan.
9. Pop the pan into the preheated oven and bake for about 25 to 30 minutes or until the egg is set.

10. Remove the pan from the oven and cool for a few minutes. Cut the prepared baked eggs into wedges and serve immediately.

11. Enjoy!

Cowboy Breakfast Skillet

Ingredients:

- 1/2 lb. breakfast sausage
- 3 eggs
- 1 medium sweet potato, diced
- 1/2 avocado, diced
- Hot sauce, to taste
- Handful cilantro
- Raw cheese, optional
- Salt, to taste
- Pepper, to taste

Instructions:

1. Crank up your oven to 400°F and allow the oven to preheat.
2. Heat an oven proof or cast iron skillet over a medium high flame and add the breakfast sausage to it. Season with salt and pepper. Crumble it while it cooks.
3. Once the sausage is well browned, remove the crumbled sausage from the pan using a slotted spoon and set aside.
4. Add the sweet potato into the grease leftover in the pan and toss well until cooked through and crispy. Season with salt and pepper.
5. Add the cooked sausage back into the pan and mix well.
6. Using the back of a round spoon make about 3 wells in the potato and sausage mix. Take the skillet off the flame.
7. Crack an egg into a well each.

8. Place the skillet into the preheated oven and bake for about 5 minutes or until the eggs are just set.

9. Switch the oven setting to broil and cook the top off the yolks for a few minutes until the eggs are firm but still runny.

10. Carefully take the pan out of the oven and top it with some chopped cilantro and some hot sauce as per your taste.

11. Serve hot by scooping the egg, along with the sausage and greens, onto a plate. Season the egg with salt and pepper if required.

12. Enjoy!

Broccoli & Cheese Mini Egg Omelets

Ingredients:

- 2 cups broccoli florets
- 1/2 cup egg whites
- 2 whole large eggs
- 2 tablespoons low fat cheddar, shredded
- 1/2 teaspoon olive oil
- 2 tablespoons grated pecorino Romano
- Salt, to taste
- Freshly cracked pepper, to taste
- Cooking spray, as required

Instructions:

1. Crank up your oven to 350 degrees F and allow the oven to preheat.
2. Pour a little water into a large vessel and place a steamer basket on it. Add the broccoli to the basket and cover. Steam for about 7 to 8 minutes or until tender.
3. Once done, crumble into smaller pieces and toss well with olive oil, pepper and salt.
4. Spray a regular cupcake tin with some cooking spray and spoon the broccoli mix into the cupcake molds.
5. Place the egg whites in a medium sized bowl. Add in the whole eggs and grated pecorino Romano. Whisk well to combine. Season with salt and pepper.

6. Pour the egg mix over the broccoli and fill until about 3/4ths of the mold is full.

7. Top the egg with some shredded cheddar.

8. Pop the cupcake tin into the preheated oven and bake for about 10 to 15 minutes or until cooked through.

9. Remove the cupcake tin from the oven and cool for a few minutes.

10. De-mold the mini egg omelets and serve immediately.

11. Enjoy!

Tex-Mex Scramble

Ingredients:

- 1/2 slice cheddar
- 3 eggs
- 1/8 cup chopped green pepper
- 1 tablespoon water
- 1/8 cup chopped red onion
- 1/4 cup frozen spinach, thawed and drained
- 1 cherry tomato, diced
- 3 jalapeno pepper slices, chopped
- 1 tablespoon salsa
- 1 tablespoon oil of your choice

Instructions:

1. Heat a cast iron skillet over a medium flame. Add in the oil and heat until lightly smoking.
2. Combine the eggs, pepper, tomatoes, jalapenos, water, onion and spinach together in a medium mixing bowl and whisk well until well combined.
3. Pour the mix onto the hot pan and cook until the eggs reach the consistency you like, stirring to scramble the egg.
4. When the eggs are just done, turn the flame off and place the cheddar cheese slice on the eggs. Cover the skillet with a lid and let it sit for about 5 minutes.
5. Serve immediately, topped with a tablespoon of salsa.
6. Enjoy!

Savory Cheese Chive Waffles

Ingredients:

- 1/2 cup raw cauliflower, processed into a fine crumb
- 1/6 cup Parmesan cheese, shredded
- 1/2 cup processed mozzarella shredded cheese
- 1 egg
- ½ tablespoon chives
- ½ teaspoon onion powder
- ½ teaspoon garlic powder
- ¼ teaspoon pepper

Instructions:

1. Prepare the waffle batter by combining all the ingredients together in a large mixing bowl. Whisk until it forms a uniformly thick batter.
2. Heat a waffle maker until heated through.
3. Pour about 1/4th of the prepared batter on the girdle. Shut the waffle maker and set the time for about 6 minutes.
4. After the fourth minute, lightly peak at the waffles cooking. If the waffle sticks, cook it for a little longer.
5. Once cooked, slowly extract the waffle from the waffle maker and cool it on the plate.
6. Serve immediately with a side of eggs cooked sunny side up.
7. Enjoy!

Swedish Breakfast Buns

Ingredients:

- 1 eggs
- 6 tablespoons almond flour
- ½ tablespoon sunflower seeds, shells removed
- ½ tablespoon whole flax seeds
- 1 tablespoon psyllium husk powder
- ¼ teaspoon salt
- ½ teaspoon baking powder
- 1 tablespoon olive oil
- ¼ cup sour cream

Instructions:

1. Crank up your oven to 400°F and allow the oven to preheat.
2. Combine the almond flour, psyllium husk, baking powder, sunflower seeds, flax seeds and salt together in a bowl.
3. In a small mixing bowl whisk together the egg, sour cream and olive oil.
4. Once combined, pour the wet ingredients into the dry ingredients and mix well to form a soft dough.
5. Cover and set aside for about 5 minutes.

6. Divide the dough into 4 equal parts and shape into smooth rounds.

7. Place the dough balls in a cake pan (a 9 inch circular cake pan should do).

8. Pop the cake pan into the preheated oven and bake for about 20 to 25 minutes, or until they are well browned.

9. Cool and serve with eggs cooked to your preference.

10. Enjoy!

Eggs Benedict with a Lazy Hollandaise Sauce

Ingredients:

- 1 egg
- 1 slice of ham
- 2 tablespoons butter
- 1 recipe Lazy Hollandaise Sauce (mentioned below)

Instructions:

1. Heat a small pan over a medium flame. Add in the butter and when well heated through, add in the egg and scramble the egg inn it. Do not scramble it too much and ensure that the egg cooks in single mass.
2. Flip the eggs over to cook the other side through. Fold once (or more than once) to create a small muffin like structure with the egg. Cool for about 3 minutes.
3. Cut the ham into a circle that will fit the diameter of the "egg muffin".
4. Place the egg muffin on the slice of ham and serve immediately topped with some hollandaise.
5. Enjoy!

Lazy Hollandaise Sauce

Ingredients:

- 1 teaspoon lemon juice
- ¼ cup mayonnaise
- 1/4 teaspoon pepper

Instructions:

1. In a small bowl blend together the mayonnaise, lemon juice and pepper together.
2. Lightly heat the sauce and your sauce is ready to serve!

Low Carb Pancake Crepes

Ingredients:

- 1/2 teaspoon butter
- 1 and 1/2 ounces cream cheese, softened
- 1/2 teaspoon ground cinnamon
- 1 egg, beaten
- 1 and 1/2 teaspoons sugar free syrup

Instructions:

1. Place the beaten egg in a medium sized bowl. Add in about one tablespoon of cream cheese and mash using the back of a spoon until smooth and lump free. Continue adding the cream cheese until it forms a smooth mixture.
2. Pour in the sugar free syrup and mix well. Add in the cinnamon and mix well.
3. Place the butter in a non-stick skillet and heat over a medium high flame. Once the butter has melted, lower the heat to a medium low and add in a few tablespoons of the prepared cream cheese and egg mix.
4. Swirl the pan until the mixture coats the bottom of the skillet. Let the batter cook untouched until it is set. It should take about 4 minutes.
5. Flip over using a spatula and cook on the other side until the crepe is lightly browned.
6. Serve immediately.
7. Enjoy!

Baby Spinach Omelet

Ingredients:

- 4 eggs
- 3 tablespoons grated Parmesan cheese
- 2 cups baby spinach leaves, torn into bite sized pieces
- 1/2 teaspoon onion powder
- Salt, to taste
- 1/4 teaspoon ground nutmeg
- Pepper, to taste

Instructions:

1. Place the eggs in a medium bowl and beat well until lightly frothy. Add in the baby spinach leaves and the grated Parmesan and mix well.
2. Add in the nutmeg, salt, onion powder and pepper. Mix well to ensure that there are now lumps of spices.
3. Spray a medium skillet with some cooking spray and heat over a medium high flame until lightly smoking.
4. Pour in the egg mixture and swirl the pan around until it coats the bottom of the skillet.
5. Cook the mixture for about 3 minutes or until it is partially set.
6. Carefully flip over the omelet using a spatula and continue cooking the egg for another 3 to 4 minutes or until set.

7. Lower the heat to medium low and let the egg cook for another 2 minutes or until it reaches the desired level of doneness.

8. Serve immediately.

9. Enjoy!

Chapter 9: Lunch / Dinner Recipes with Low Carb

Ground Beef With Sliced Bell Peppers

Ingredients:

- 1 tablespoon Coconut Oil
- 1 Onion, finely chopped
- ½ lb. Ground Beef
- ½ cup Spinach, thinly sliced
- 1 bell pepper, thinly sliced
- Salt, to taste
- Pepper, to taste
- Cayenne, to taste

Instructions:

1. Pour the coconut oil into a pan and heat on a medium high flame until heated through.
2. Add in the onion and cook until the onion is translucent.
3. Once the onion is cooked, add in the ground beef and mix well until well browned.
4. Season with spices according to taste.
5. Top with the spinach and belle pepper and cook uncovered, constantly stirring until cooked through.
6. Serve hot.
7. Enjoy!

Bacon Wrapped Mini Meatloaves

Ingredients:

- 1/2 lb. ground beef
- 4 additional strips of bacon
- 1/4 lb. bacon, cut in small chunks
- 2 tablespoons coconut milk
- 3 tablespoons fresh chives, minced
- 1 garlic clove, minced
- Fresh parsley, chopped
- Freshly ground black pepper, to taste
- Salt, to taste

Instructions:

1. Crank up your oven to 400 degrees F and allow the oven to preheat.
2. Combine the ground beef, garlic, coconut milk, bacon chunks and chives together in a large mixing bowl using a wooden spoon or an electric mixer. Keep mixing until the ingredients hold together.
3. Season with salt and pepper to taste. (Use a low amount of salt as the bacon is already salted)
4. In a medium sized muffin tin, place the bacon on the sides of the mold.
5. Fill the same four molds with the prepared beef mixture.

6. Pop the muffin tray into the preheated oven and bake for about 30 to 35 minutes.

7. Once cooked through, remove the muffin tin from the oven and cool for about 10 minutes or until the muffins are cool enough to handle.

8. De-mold the mini meatloaves and serve immediately topped with some fresh parsley.

9. Enjoy!

Low Carb Lettuce Wraps

Ingredients:

- 1 ½ tablespoons fat of your choice, preferably olive oil or coconut oil
- 2 oz. shiitake mushrooms, chopped
- 1/2 lb. boneless and skinless chicken breasts, chopped into tiny cubes
- 1/4 onion diced
- 1 green onion, finely chopped
- 2 cloves garlic, minced
- Handful of cilantro, chopped
- 2 tablespoons low sodium soy sauce
- Juice of ½ lemon
- ½ teaspoon chili garlic sauce
- Iceberg lettuce
- ½ teaspoon sesame oil
- ½ avocado, sliced

Instructions:

1. Place about 1 tablespoon of the fat of your choice in a small sauté pan and heat on a medium low flame until lightly smoking.
2. Add the chicken to the pan and toss well until cooked through.

3. While the chicken is sizzling in the pan, place the lemon juice, soy sauce, green onion, chili garlic sauce, sesame oil and cilantro together in a mixing bowl.

4. Once the chicken is done, add it to the bowl and mix well.

5. While the chicken cooks, add the chili sauce, lemon juice, sesame oil, soy sauce, green onions and cilantro into a serving bowl.

6. Once the chicken is done, add it to the bowl.

7. Add the remaining fat to the sauté pan and heat. Once smoking, add in the onion, mushrooms and garlic to it. Sauté for about 10 minutes or until cooked through.

8. Empty the contents of the sauté pan into the mixing bowl and toss well to coat.

9. Carefully cut away the stem of the lettuce. Remove individual lettuce leaves and wash well.

10. Make small "cups" out of the lettuce and spoon some of the prepared chicken filling into the lettuce cup.

11. Serve immediately topped with a slice of avocado.

12. Enjoy!

Delicious Chili Cheese Dogs

Ingredients:

- 1 ½ sweet potatoes, cut into halves length wise
- 3 low fat, low sodium hot dogs
- 2 tablespoons Olive oil + oil for dousing sweet potatoes
- ½ lb. ground beef
- 1 Chipotle pepper soaked in adobe sauce, chopped
- ½ 15 oz. can fire roasted tomatoes, drained out of the liquid, chopped finely
- ¼ red onion, diced
- ½ tablespoon chili powder
- 1 clove of garlic, minced
- ¼ teaspoon cocoa powder (optional)
- Pepper, to taste
- Salt, to taste
- 1 ½ oz. sharp cheddar cheese, grated

Instructions:

1. Crank up your oven to 450 degrees F and allow the oven to preheat.
2. Douse your sweet potato halves with a healthy amount of olive oil. Place the oil-covered sweet potatoes on a baking sheet with their skin side up.

3. Pop the baking sheet into the preheated oven and bake for about 30 minutes or until the skin is crispy and the insides soften.

4. While the sweet potatoes bake, add 2 tablespoons olive oil into a sauté pan. Hat on a medium low flame until lightly smoking.

5. Add in the onions and garlic and sauté for about 10 minutes or until softened.

6. Add in the tomatoes, cocoa powder, chipotle peppers, chili powder, salt and pepper. Mix well to combine.

7. Crumble the ground beef into the pan, ensuring there are no large chunks of ground beef in the pan. Continue cooking the chili until all the components of the chili are cooked thoroughly.

8. Once the sweet potatoes are cooked, remove them from the baking sheet. Place the hot dogs on the baking sheet and pop them into the still hot oven for about 7 minutes.

9. Spoon out the mushy center of the sweet potatoes and save the sweet potato mush for future use.

10. To assemble your Chili Cheese Dogs place the crisp sweet potato skins on a serving plate. Place the hot dog on the crispy skin, spoon some prepared chili onto it and sprinkle some grated cheese over the chili.

11. Serve immediately.

12. Enjoy!

Crispy Carnitas

Ingredients:

- ½ onion, chopped or thinly sliced
- 2 pounds pork shoulder, cut into 5 pieces
- ½ teaspoon cumin
- ¾ teaspoon salt
- ½ teaspoon chili powder
- 1 bay leaf
- ½ cinnamon stick
- 2 garlic cloves, thinly sliced
- Water, for braising

Instructions:

1. Crank up your oven to 350 °F and allow the oven to preheat.
2. Combine the cumin, salt and chili powder together to make a spice rub. Rub it well onto the pork shoulder pieces.
3. In a large heavy bottomed pot, place the spice rubbed meat pieces along with the cinnamon stick, garlic, bay leaf and the onion. Try to make sure that your meat is in a single layer.
4. Pour some water over the meat, until the water level is almost, but not completely, covering the meat.
5. Place the pot into the oven uncovered and allow to braise for about 3 ½ to 4 hours. You will know your meat is

cooked when it becomes extremely tender, browns and most of the braising liquid is gone.

6. Once the meat is cooked, carefully remove the pot from the oven. Using tongs remove the meat pieces onto a large cutting board and let it cool a bit, before slicing it into thin slices or shredding it using your hands.

7. Remove the bay leaf and cinnamon stick from the pot and add the thinly sliced or shredded meat into the pot. Return the pot into the oven.

8. Let the meat roast in the oven, stirring it with a wooden spoon occasionally, until the meat is crispy and becomes really dark. (If you wish to speed up the process, spread the meat and the liquid from the pot into a baking sheet and spread it into a single even layer. The meat will become crisp faster.)

9. Serve the crisp meat with low carb bread.

10. Enjoy!

Pizza Topping Casserole

Ingredients:

- 2 tablespoons olive oil
- ½ pound bulk Italian sausage, chopped into bite sized pieces
- 2 eggs
- 4 ounces fresh mushrooms, sliced
- ¼ cup heavy cream
- ¼ teaspoon garlic powder
- 2 tablespoons low sodium pizza sauce
- ¼ teaspoon Italian seasoning
- ¼ cup green pepper, chopped
- 2 ounces pepperoni, chopped
- 4 ounces whole milk mozzarella cheese, cubed
- Crushed red pepper, optional
- ¼ cup red onion, cut into thin slices

Instructions:

1. Heat the olive oil in a sauté pan and heat over a medium high flame until lightly smoking. Add in the sausage and mushrooms and cook until the meat is well browned and the mushrooms are cooked through.

2. Place the eggs, pizza sauce, garlic powder, Italian seasoning, crushed red pepper and cream in a medium bowl. Whisk well to combine.

3. Grease a 7 x 12 inch shallow baking dish with some oil. Place the meats, peppers, mushrooms and mozzarella

cubes in it. Pour the prepared egg mixture over it and mix well to combine.

4. Top with the sliced red onion.

5. Sprinkle a little more garlic powder, crushed red pepper flakes and Italian seasoning over the red onion.

6. Pop the baking dish into an oven and bake at 350 degrees F for 45 to 60 minutes or until the top is well browned and a skewer inserted in the center comes out almost clean.

7. Remove the pan from the oven and let it stand for about 5 minutes before cutting into bite sized pieces.

8. Serve hot.

9. Enjoy!

Carolina Style Barbeque Meatballs

Ingredients:

<u>For the meatballs</u>

- ¼ lb. ground pork
- ¼ teaspoon granulated sugar substitute (honey for Paleo)
- ¼ teaspoon paprika (smoked if you have it)
- ¼ teaspoon salt
- ¼ teaspoon black pepper
- ¼ teaspoon cayenne pepper
- ¼ teaspoon ground cumin
- ¼ teaspoon celery salt
- ¼ egg
- 2 tablespoons almond flour
- ½ tablespoon water

<u>For the low carb BBQ sauce</u>

- 2 tablespoons yellow mustard
- ½ teaspoon Hot Sauce
- ¼ tablespoon dried onion flakes
- 1 tablespoon honey
- ¼ tablespoon apple cider vinegar
- ¼ tablespoon low sugar ketchup
- Salt, to taste
- Pepper, to taste

Instructions:

For the low carb BBQ sauce

1. Place all the ingredients of the sauce in a small saucepan and mix well until well combined.
2. Heat over a low flame for about 8 minutes until simmering.

For the meatballs

1. Combine all the ingredients for the meatballs in a medium sized mixing bowl until well combined. Divide the meatball mix into 4 equal parts and form into smooth balls.
2. Heat a little oil in a large non-stick frying pan and lightly fry the meatballs until well browned and cooked through. It should take about 4 minutes per side to cook.
3. Douse the meatballs in the prepared barbeque sauce and spread the sauce and meatballs onto a parchment lined baking sheet. Broil for about 3 to 4 minutes.
4. Serve hot with some low carb coleslaw.
5. Enjoy!

Cheese Enchiladas

Ingredients:

<u>For the Enchiladas</u>

- 1 ½ cups frozen cauliflower, thawed, drained and processed / diced
- 2 eggs, well beaten
- 1 ½ cups mozzarella, grated

<u>For the Enchilada Sauce</u>

- ¼ cup onion, chopped
- 1 large clove of garlic, chopped or crushed
- ½ tablespoon chili powder
- 2 tablespoons extra virgin olive oil
- ½ teaspoon oregano
- 1 teaspoon cumin
- ½ teaspoon salt
- 1/4 teaspoon pepper
- ½ cup pizza sauce or low sugar tomato sauce
- 1 cup Cheddar Cheese, shredded
- 1 cup Monterey Jack or Pepper Jack, shredded

Instructions:

<u>For the Enchiladas</u>

1. Crank up the oven to 450 degrees F and allow the oven to preheat.

2. Combine the processed cauliflower, grated cheese and eggs together in a mixing bowl.

3. Grease a cookie sheet and pour about 1/3 cup of the dough into 6, 6-inch rounds. Place the cookie sheet into the preheated oven and bake for about 15 minutes or until the edges of the shell brown and the whole crust has a golden hue to it.

4. Remove the shells from the oven and cool the shells before loosening the shells from the pan.

5. Once the shell is set, place the shell aside.

For the Enchilada Sauce

1. Crank up the oven to 350 degrees F and allow the oven to preheat.

2. Pour the oil into a saucepan and heat on a medium high flame until lightly smoking. Add the garlic, onion and chili powder to it and sauté for about 5 minutes or until tender.

3. Add in the oregano, salt, pizza sauce, cumin, and pepper to the pan and mix well. Keep mixing until the sauce is heated through.

4. Add in about half the cheeses and mix well.

5. Take the prepared shells and dip into the heated enchilada sauce.

6. Place the sauce dipped shells, golden size up, onto an ungreased 9 x 13 inch casserole dish.

7. Spoon about 2 tablespoons of the remaining cheeses into the shells and roll into a tight roll. Place the enchiladas, seam side down and top with the remaining enchilada sauce.

8. Pop into the oven and bake for about 20 to 25 minutes until the cheese is gooey and bubbly.

9. Serve immediately.

10. Enjoy!

Swedish Meatballs

Ingredients:

- ½ teaspoon olive oil
- 1 clove garlic, minced
- ½ small onion, minced
- ½ celery stalk, minced
- ½ lb. 93% lean ground beef
- 2 tablespoons minced parsley
- 1 small egg
- Salt, to taste
- 2 tablespoons seasoned breadcrumbs
- Pepper, to taste
- 1 cup reduced sodium beef stock
- ¼ teaspoon allspice
- 1 oz. light cream cheese

Instructions:

1. Pour the oil into a deep sauté pan and heat over a medium high flame. Add in the onion and garlic and sauté until the garlic is aromatic and the onion is translucent. This should take about 5 minutes.

2. Add in the parsley and celery and cook for another 4 to 5 minutes, or until tender. Allow the sautéed vegetables to cool slightly.

3. Combine the beef, sautéed vegetable mixture, salt, allspice, egg, breadcrumbs and pepper together in a large mixing bowl. Mix well.

4. Scoop out about 2 tablespoons of the meatball mix and form into a smooth meatball.

5. Pour the beef stock into a pan and heat on a high flame until bubbling. Reduce the heat to a medium low and slowly put the meatballs into the pan.

6. Cover the pan with a lid and cook for about 20 minutes.

7. Using a slotted spoon, drain the meatballs from the broth and place on a serving dish.

8. Strain the stock and pour into a blender jar. Add in the cream cheese and pulse until it forms a smooth mix.

9. Return the broth and cream cheese mix into the pan and simmer the sauce until it thickens.

10. Pour the sauce over the prepared meatballs and serve immediately with toothpicks or over some gluten free noodles.

11. Enjoy!

Honey Mustard Cuban Pork Burgers

Ingredients:

- ½ pound ground pork breakfast sausage
- 1 egg white, whisked
- ½ cup plantain chips
- 1 ½ tablespoons bacon fat
- ½ teaspoon garlic powder
- 1 garlic clove, minced
- Salt, to taste
- ½ avocado, sliced
- Pepper, to taste
- ½ tablespoon raw honey
- ½ teaspoon yellow mustard
- ½ teaspoon Dijon mustard
- Arugula, to garnish

Instructions:

1. Crank your oven to 350 degrees F and allow the oven to preheat.
2. In jar of a food processor, place the plantain chips and pulse until it gets a coarse breadcrumb like consistency.
3. Divide the meat into two halves and make 2 burger patties out of it.

4. Whisk the egg white using a wire whisk or an electric blender until it is bubbly. Place the plantain breadcrumbs in another bowl.

5. Dip each burger patty into the whisked egg white and in the plantain mixture, until well coated. Sprinkle a pinch of salt, garlic powder and pepper over both sides of the burger patty.

6. Heat a cast iron skillet over a medium high flame and add the bacon fat to it. Add in the minced garlic cloves and cook the garlic until aromatic.

7. Add the burger patties to the skillet and cook for about 4 minutes on each side, ensuring that the plantain chips don't burn.

8. After the burger patties have been fried, place the skillet into the preheated oven and cook for about 8 to 10 minutes or until the burger patties are cooked to your preference.

9. While the burgers are in the oven, place the honey, Dijon mustard and yellow mustard together in a small mixing bowl. Whisk well until well combined.

10. Once the burger patties are cooked, rest the, for 2 minutes before serving.

11. Top the patties with a slice of avocado and the prepared honey mustard dressing.

12. Serve immediately garnished with some arugula.

13. Enjoy!

Asian Inspired Chicken Wings

Ingredients:

- 2 tablespoons coconut oil
- 1 ½ pounds chicken wings, separated
- 2 cloves fresh garlic, chopped
- 1 tablespoon sesame oil
- 1 tablespoon extra-virgin coconut oil
- ½ tablespoon fresh ginger, chopped
- ½ teaspoon fennel seed
- ½ teaspoon anise seed
- 2 tablespoons coconut aminos (or if unavailable, use reduced sodium tamari soy sauce)
- 1 tablespoon coconut vinegar (or if unavailable, use apple cider vinegar)
- 1 tablespoon honey
- ½ tablespoon fish sauce

Instructions:

1. Pat dry the chicken wings with a paper towel and place them in a large bowl.
2. Place the coconut oil in a small saucepan and heat over a medium high flame.

3. Add the chopped ginger, anise seed, garlic and fennel seeds into the saucepan and cook, stirring constantly to ensure that they don't burn.

4. Keep cooking until the contents of the saucepan are fragrant. It should take about 2 to 3 minutes.

5. Add in the coconut aminos (or the reduced sodium tamari soy sauce), coconut vinegar (or the apple cider vinegar), honey and the fish sauce to the pan and bring to a boil.

6. Once bubbling, reduce the flame and let it simmer for a minute.

7. Remove the pan off the heat and mix in the sesame oil.

8. Pour the prepared mix over the chicken wings in the bowl and mix well to coat.

9. Once the chicken wings have cooled down enough to be handled, cover the chicken wings and let them marinate in the fridge overnight. Mix them around once or twice so that they are evenly treated.

10. Remove the extra marinade from the wings and place on a smoldering hot grill. Barbeque the wings for about 20 minutes or until the wings are cooked to perfection on both sides.

11. If you do not have a grill, you can place the marinated wings on a lined baking sheet and pop into a preheated oven and bake for an hour at 375 degrees F. or until cooked through.

12. Serve with your favorite low carb condiment.

13. Enjoy!

Bora Bora Fireballs

Ingredients:

- ¾ cup unsweetened shredded coconut
- ¼ teaspoon plus ¼ teaspoon salt
- ¾ teaspoon plus ½ teaspoon ground cayenne pepper
- ½ cup canned crushed pineapple, packed in its juice, sugar free
- 1 tablespoon coconut aminos or homemade substitute
- ¾ teaspoons dried ginger
- 2 cloves garlic, minced (about ½ tablespoon)
- 2 scallions, very thinly sliced, white and green (about 2 tablespoons)
- ¼ fresh jalapeño, ribs and seeds removed, finely minced (about 1 teaspoon)
- 1 large egg, lightly beaten
- 1 pound ground pork

Instructions:

1. Crank up the oven to 375 degrees F and allow the oven to preheat.
2. Line a large baking sheet with some heavy-duty foil or some parchment paper. Set aside.
3. Place a large non-stick skillet on a medium high flame and heat thoroughly. Add in the coconut and dry roast it for 3 to 4 minutes, or until well browned.

4. Remove the coconut from the skillet and add in the ½ teaspoon salt and ¾ teaspoon cayenne. Mix well and place it aside until cooled.

5. Place the pineapple in a sieve with a bowl under it and collect the juice in the bowl. Using the back of a wooden spoon, press the pineapple against the sieve to crush it and release the excess moisture. Set the juice aside.

6. Transfer the crushed pineapple into a large mixing bowl and add ½ teaspoon salt, coconut aminos, garlic, jalapeno, the remaining cayenne, ginger, scallions and eggs. Mix well to combine.

7. Add the pork to the bowl, slowly crumbling it with your hands and knead with your hands until all the ingredients are properly incorporated.

8. Measure out about a tablespoon of the meatball mix and makes a smooth ball with it. Repeat with the remaining meatball mix.

9. Dip it into the bowl of pineapple juice and then roll it into the seasoned coconut mix.

10. Place the prepared meatballs onto the prepared baking sheet, with about ½ an inch between two meatballs.

11. Pop the baking sheet into the preheated oven and bake for about 30 to 40 minutes until the meatballs are golden brown.

12. Serve with some Sunshine sauce.

13. Enjoy!

Simple Herb Crusted Salmon

Ingredients:

For the salmon

- 1 salmon fillet (about 6 oz.)
- ½ heaping tablespoon coconut flour
- 1 tablespoon fresh parsley
- ½ tablespoon olive oil
- ½ tablespoon Dijon mustard
- Salt, to taste
- Pepper, to taste

For the salad

- 1 cups arugula
- ¼ red onion, sliced thin
- Juice of ½ lemon
- ½ tablespoon white wine vinegar
- ½ tablespoon olive oil
- Salt, to taste
- Pepper, to taste

Instructions

1. Crank up the oven to 450 degrees F and allow the oven to preheat.
2. Line a baking sheet with heavy-duty aluminum foil or parchment paper and place the salmon fillet on it.
3. Rub the olive oil and Dijon mustard on the salmon using your fingers.

4. Combine the parsley, coconut flour, salt and pepper together in a small mixing bowl.

5. Spoon the prepared toppings onto the salmon and pat the topping onto the salmon using your fingers.

6. Pop the baking sheet into the preheated oven and cook for about 15 to 20 minutes or until your salmon is cooked to your preference.

7. While the salmon is cooking, combine all the ingredients for the salad together in a large mixing bowl. Toss well until the ingredients are well combined.

8. When the salmon is cooked, spoon the salad onto a serving plate and place the oven baked salmon fillet on it.

9. Serve immediately.

10. Enjoy!

Buttery Catfish In A Creamy Shallot Sauce

Ingredients:

- 1 catfish fillet (about ½ pound of fish)
- ½ tablespoon olive oil
- ½ shallot, finely chopped
- 1 ½ tablespoons butter
- 1/4 cup coconut milk
- Juice from ½ lemon
- Finely chopped chives for garnish

Instructions:

1. Using a paper towel, pat dry the fish and lightly sprinkle salt over the fillet and rub it lightly using your fingers.
2. Pour the olive oil into a medium sized skillet and heat over a medium high flame until lightly smoking. Add the shallots to the pan and cook for about 30 seconds.
3. Add the butter to the pan and heat gently until the butter has completely melted.
4. Add in the fish fillet and allow it to fry untouched for about 5 minutes. Flip and cook the other side for another 5 minutes.
5. Remove the fish from the skillet and set aside.
6. Lower the heat and add the lemon juice to the skillet.
7. Lightly scrape the leftover bits of fish in the pan and pour in the coconut milk.

8. Simmer the coconut milk for about 3 minutes, giving it an occasional stir, until the sauce thickens.

9. Pour the prepared sauce over the fried fish and top with some chives.

10. Serve hot.

11. Enjoy!

Cheesy Tuna Casserole

Ingredients:

- 1 6-ounce can tuna, drained
- 8 ounces frozen green beans, French cut
- 2 ounces fresh mushrooms, chopped (about 5 mushrooms)
- ½ stalk celery, finely chopped
- 1 tablespoon onion, finely chopped
- 1 tablespoon butter
- 2 tablespoons chicken broth
- ½ cup heavy cream
- Salt, to taste
- Pepper, to taste
- Xanthan gum, optional
- 2 ounces cheddar cheese, shredded

Instructions:

1. Place the green beans in a medium sized pot and cook them according to the instructions on the package. Drain well.
2. While the green beans cook, heat the butter in the pan and add in the mushrooms, onion and celery. Sauté the vegetables until they are soft and are starting to brown around the edges.

3. Pour in the broth and heat on a high flame until it starts boiling. Reduce the flame to a medium low when the liquid is reduced to almost half its original quantity and in the cream and mix well to combine. Increase the flame to high again and let it boil.

4. Turn the heat down to a medium low and let the sauce cook until it thickens. Stir frequently to ensure that it doesn't boil over. Season the sauce to taste.

5. Combine the tuna, mushroom sauce and the green beans together. Taste and season to taste.

6. Add in the cheese and mix well.

7. Pour the prepared mix into a 2-quart casserole.

8. Pop the casserole into an oven or microwave and cook until the cheese melts and is gooey and bubbly.

9. Cool for a bit and serve with a fresh salad.

10. Enjoy!

Roasted Salmon and Vegetables with Coconut Aminos

Ingredients:

- 1/4 cup coconut aminos or tamari
- 1 tablespoon coconut oil or olive oil
- 1 tablespoon toasted sesame oil
- 3 green onions, roughly chopped
- 4 (6-ounce) salmon fillets
- 2 to 4 cloves of garlic
- 3/4 pound green beans
- 3 red bell peppers, thinly sliced, deseeded
- 1 pound mushrooms, roughly chopped
- Sea salt, to taste
- Freshly ground black pepper, to taste

Instructions:

1. Crank up the oven to 450 degrees F and allow the oven to preheat for a while.
2. Line three baking pans with heavy-duty aluminum foil and place in the oven to heat. (One pan is for the salmon fillets and the other two will be for the vegetables).
3. Place the coconut aminos (or the tamari), sesame oil, coconut oil or olive oil, garlic and green onions in the jar of

the blender and blitz for about 30 seconds or until the garlic and green onions are finely chopped.

4. Set aside about 1 tablespoon of the prepared sauce in a small bowl and spoon the some of the remaining sauce onto the salmon pieces. Make sure to save some for the vegetables.

5. In a large bowl, combine the green beans, mushrooms and bell peppers.

6. Pour the remaining sauce over the vegetables and toss well until well coated.

7. Carefully take the hot pans out from the oven. Place the salmon pieces in a single layer in one pan. Spread the remaining vegetables in the other two pans in a single layer.

8. Pop the pans bake into the preheated oven and bake for about 10 to 15 minutes or until the salmon pieces reach the desired level of doneness.

9. Sprinkle some freshly black ground pepper and the sea salt on the pieces of sauce-coated salmon and the sauce-coated veggies.

10. Spoon the veggies onto a serving plate and place a piece of salmon over it.

11. Serve immediately with a side of tamari or coconut aminos, if required.

12. Enjoy!

Basic Buttery Baked Salmon

Ingredients:

- 1 pound salmon fillet, thawed if frozen (can use other fish too)
- Garlic powder, to taste
- 2 - 4 tablespoons butter, softened
- Salt, to taste
- Pepper, to taste

Instructions:

1. Crank up the oven to 425 degrees F and allow the oven to preheat for a few minutes.
2. Line a baking dish with some heavy-duty aluminum foil. Lightly grease the foil and place salmon fillets on it.
3. Sprinkle some garlic powder, salt and pepper over the fillets, and place the butter on the fillets. Using a pastry brush spread the butter over the fillets.
4. Pop the baking sheet into the preheated oven and bake for about 12 to 15 minutes or until the thickest part of the fillet is just done.
5. If you wish to brown the fish, broil for a couple of minutes.
6. If desired, put the fish under the broiler for a few minutes to brown the top.
7. Serve hot with your favorite low carb condiment on the side.
8. Enjoy!

Quick & Easy Low Carb Fish Sticks

Ingredients:

- 1 lb. haddock (or any other meaty white fish which is firm)
- 5 oz. of plantain chips
- Fat of your choice, ideally coconut oil or palm oil

Instructions:

1. Place the plantain chips in the jar of a food processor and process until the chips have a coarse breadcrumb like consistency.
2. Pour the coarse plantain crush into a zip lock bag and some salt to it, if your chips are unsalted.
3. Slice the fish into fillets or sticks.
4. Add a few fillets or sticks to the zip lock bag at a time, and shake the bag around the fish fillets or sticks are well coated.
5. Place the fat of your choice in a medium sized sauté pan and heat over a medium low flame until lightly smoking.
6. Place the plantain chip coated fish fillets or sticks into the hot oil and fry them on each side until golden brown. It should take a minute or less for each side of the fish.
7. Serve hot with a side of low carb condiment of your choice.
8. Enjoy!

Roasted Eggplant Salad with Goat Cheese

Ingredients:

- 1/8 cup finely chopped scallions
- 1 large eggplant, about 1 pound
- 3 tablespoons olive oil
- Kosher salt, as required
- 1 tablespoons cider vinegar
- 1/2 teaspoon smoked paprika
- 1/2 tablespoon honey
- 1/4 teaspoon cumin
- 1 tablespoon lemon juice
- 2 large garlic cloves, roughly chopped
- 1/2 tablespoon soy sauce
- 1/4 cup smoked almonds, roughly chopped
- 1/2 cup flat parsley leaves, roughly chopped
- 1 ounce goat cheese, crumbled and divided

Instructions:

1. Crank up the oven to 400 degrees F and let the oven preheat for a while.
2. Chop the eggplant into 1-inch cubes and place in a large mixing bowl. Sprinkle some kosher salt over the eggplant cubes and mix well. Set aside.
3. Combine the olive oil, honey, cumin, cider vinegar and smoked paprika together in a small bowl. Whisk well to

combine. Lightly pat dry the eggplant cubes and pour in the prepared marinade. Toss well until well coated. Add in the garlic and mix.

4. Line a large baking sheet with some parchment paper and spread the marinated eggplant on it in a single layer. Place the baking sheet in the middle rack of the preheated oven and roast for about 45 to 50 minutes or until the eggplant is tender and slightly browned around the edges. Check the eggplant around the 30-minute mark to ensure that it isn't burning! Remove the tray from the oven and cool for a few minutes.

5. In a small bowl combine the lemon juice and soy sauce together. Whisk well to combine.

6. Empty the roasted eggplant from the baking tray into a large bowl and add in the prepared lemon and soy sauce mix. Add in the parsley leaves, goat cheese (reserving some for garnishing) and the smoked almonds. Toss well to combine.

7. Transfer the finished salad into a serving bowl and serve immediately topped with the reserved crumbled goat cheese and chopped scallion.

8. Enjoy!

Portobello Mushroom Burgers

Ingredients:

- 2 Portobello mushroom caps
- 1 tablespoon olive oil
- 2 tablespoons balsamic vinegar
- 1/2 teaspoon dried basil
- 1 1/2 teaspoons minced garlic
- 1/2 teaspoon dried oregano
- Salt, to taste
- 2 (1 ounce) slices provolone cheese
- Pepper, to taste

Instructions:

1. In a shallow dish, place the Portobello mushroom caps with their rough side down.
2. Combine together oil, oregano, salt, vinegar, basil and pepper together in a small bowl. Whisk well until well combined.
3. Pour this marinade over the mushroom caps and set aside for about 20 minutes, turning over twice. Do not refrigerate.
4. Heat the grill on the medium high setting.
5. Lightly drizzle some oil on the grate. Place the marinated mushrooms on the grill. Do not throw away the leftover marinade, as it will be required for basting.

6. Grill for about 7 to 10 minutes on each side or until the Portobello caps are tender. Regularly brush the marinade onto the mushroom caps to prevent drying.

7. In the last two minutes of grilling, turn over the mushroom caps so that their smooth side is facing down and place the provolone cheese slices on them.

8. Once the cheese has melted, transfer the grilled mushroom caps onto a serving plate and serve with a side of fresh vegetables tossed with a low carb dressing.

9. Enjoy!

Chapter 10: Dessert Recipes with Low Carb

Three Minute Chocolate Cake

Ingredients:

- 2 tablespoons almond flour, ½ ounce
- ½ tablespoon cocoa
- 1/4 teaspoon baking powder
- 1 ½ tablespoons plus ½ teaspoon granulated Splenda or sugar substitute
- 1 tablespoon butter, melted
- ½ tablespoon water
- 1 egg

Instructions:

1. Combine the almond flour, baking powder, cocoa and granulated splenda into a 2 cup measuring cup.
2. Pour in the butter, egg and water. Mix well using a fork or a small wire whisk.
3. Using a spatula, scrape the sides of the cup and make sure the batter is even.
4. Cover the cup with a plastic wrap and cut a small vent on the top of it.
5. Microwave the cake on the HIGH setting for 1 minute or until the top is just set.
6. Cool the cake slightly and serve it warm topped with some whipped cream or frosting of your choice.
7. Enjoy!

Magically Moist Almond Cake

Ingredients:

- ½ cup butter, softened
- ½ cup granular Splenda or any other sugar substitute
- 2 eggs
- 1/4 cup heavy cream
- ½ teaspoon vanilla
- ¾ cup almond flour
- ¼ cup coconut flour, sifted
- ¼ teaspoon salt
- 1 teaspoon baking powder
- ½ cup water, optional

Instructions:

1. Crank up the oven to 350 degrees F and allow the oven to preheat.
2. Place all the ingredients in a large mixing bowl and whisk well using a hand mixer or an electronic mixer until it forms a smooth and creamy batter.
3. If you find the batter to be too stiff, just beat in the ½ cup of water and continue beating until well blended.
4. Grease a 9 x 13 inch pan and line it with a parchment sheet.
5. Pour the batter into the prepared pan and lightly bang it against the kitchen counter to ensure that there are no air bubbles.

6. Pop the baking dish into the preheated oven and bake for about 35 to 40 minutes or till a skewer inserted in the center of the cake comes clean and the cake is firm to touch.

7. Cool the cake in the pan before removing it from the pan. Cool on a wire rack till it cools.

8. Serve topped with some coconut cream.

9. Enjoy!

Simple Blueberry Lemon Birthday Cake

Ingredients:

<u>For the cake(s)</u>

1. 6 tablespoons coconut flour, sifted
2. 3 eggs
3. 3 tablespoons coconut milk
4. 2 tablespoons cup raw honey
5. 1 teaspoon vanilla extract
6. Juice of 1 lemon
7. ½ teaspoon lemon zest
8. ¼ teaspoon baking soda
9. Pinch of salt
10. ¼ cup fresh blueberries
11. 1 tablespoon coconut oil (to grease the pans)

<u>For the frosting</u>

- ¼ cup coconut cream concentrate, melted
- Juice of ½ lemon
- 1/8 cup raw honey

Instructions:

1. Crank up the oven to 350 degrees F and allow the oven to preheat for a while.
2. Sieve the coconut flour into a bowl, making sure that there are no clumps in the coconut flour.

3. Pour the almond milk and egg into the bowl with the coconut flour and whisk well using a wire whisk or an electronic beater, until it forms a smooth batter.

4. Add in the honey, lemon juice, baking soda, vanilla extract lemon zest and salt to it. Fold until well combined.

5. Lightly dust the blueberries with some icing sugar and add them to the batter.

6. Fold them in carefully, ensuring that they don't get bruised or muddled in the process.

7. Pour the coconut oil into two spring form tins and grease well.

8. Distribute the batter in even parts on the two greased tins and place on a baking sheet so that there is even baking.

9. Pop the baking sheet into the preheated oven and bake it for about 40 to 45 minutes or till a skewer inserted in the center of the cake comes out clean and the cake is firm to touch.

10. Remove the baking sheet from the oven and cool the cakes in the pan for a few minutes before transferring them to a wire rack to cool.

11. While the cakes cool, combine the melted coconut butter, honey and lemon juice together and whisk well to combine.

12. Transfer the cakes onto serving plates and pour the prepared frosting over them.

13. Serve immediately.

14. Enjoy!

Simply Delicious Sugar Free Cheesecake

Ingredients:

<u>For the Filling:</u>

- 2 ½ 8-ounce packages cream cheese, softened
- ¾ cup sugar equivalent substitute
- 2 eggs
- ¼ cup Plain Greek yogurt
- ½ tablespoon lemon juice
- ¾ teaspoon vanilla extract

<u>For the crust:</u>

- ½ cup almonds, whole
- 1 tablespoon sugar equivalent substitute
- 2 tablespoons butter, melted

<u>For the topping:</u>

- ½ cup unsweetened, heavy whipping cream
- 1 tablespoon sugar equivalent substitute
- Fresh fruit

Instructions:

<u>For the crust:</u>

1. Place the nuts in the food processor and pulse until it is coarse and has a crushed graham cracker like feel.
2. Add in the almond meal, sweetener and butter to the pulsed nuts and mix well.

3. Press the blend into the bottom of a 10-inch spring form pan and let it freeze.

For the Filling:

1. Crank up the oven to 325 degrees F and allow the oven to preheat for a while.
2. Place the cream cheese and the sweetener in the bowl of a stand mixer. Beat on a medium speed for about a minute.
3. Once smooth, reduce the speed to low and add in the eggs one at a time until it is just combined.
4. Once done, add in the yogurt, vanilla extract and lemon juice and beat for another 20 seconds at the most.
5. Pour the prepared filling onto the frozen crust.
6. Place the spring form tin in the preheated oven with a pan of water in the pan below it.
7. Bake for about 90 to 105 minutes (about 1 hour 15 minutes to 1 hour 30 minutes).
8. Remove the cheesecake from the oven and cool for about 10 minutes before transferring the cheesecake into the refrigerator to chill.

For the topping:

1. To prepare the topping combine the sweetener and whipping cream and beat for about 5 to 7 minutes or until it forms stiff peaks.
2. Frost the top of the cheesecake with the prepared frosting and cover it with fresh fruit.
3. Serve immediately.
4. Enjoy!

Almond Coconut Bars

Ingredients:

- 1/2 cup Shredded Unsweetened Coconut
- 1 cup whole Raw Almonds
- 1/4 cup Almond Butter
- 6 tablespoons extra virgin coconut oil
- ½ tablespoon Coconut Flour
- ¼ teaspoon Salt
- ¾ tablespoon Blackstrap Molasses
- ½ tablespoon Vanilla Extract
- 1 ½ oz. 80% Dark Chocolate

Instructions:

1. Place the coconut oil into a small bowl and heat in a microwave over a low power until melted.
2. Place a heavy-duty foil or wax paper in a 9 x 9 inch pan.
3. Place the almonds in the food processor and pulse until it gets the texture of coarse sand.
4. Add in all the ingredients, except the chocolate, to the food processor and blitz until it forms a coarse paste.
5. Pour the prepared mix into the lined tin and make sure it forms a smooth even layer. Pop the tin into the refrigerator and chill for at least an hour.
6. While it cools, heat the chocolate and melt it over a double boiler until liquefied.

7. Pour the melted chocolate over the almond base using a spoon or a spatula until it forms an even layer.

8. Place the tin back into the refrigerator and chill for at least 10 minutes or until the chocolate is solid but still a little soft in the center.

9. Cut the almond bars into small rectangles and serve or store in a sealed container in the fridge.

10. Enjoy!

Chocolate "Peanut Butter" Ice Cream with Chocolate Shell

Ingredients:

For the ice cream

- 1 (14 ounce) can coconut milk
- 1 ½ tablespoons unsweetened cocoa powder
- ⅓ cup raw honey
- ½ teaspoon instant coffee
- ¼ teaspoon cinnamon
- Pinch of salt
- ¼ cup sunflower seed butter (or other nut butter)

For the chocolate shell

- 2 tablespoons coconut oil, melted
- ½ tablespoon unsweetened cocoa powder
- ½ tablespoon sunflower seed butter (or other nut butter)
- ½ tablespoon raw honey
- ¼ teaspoon vanilla extract
- Pinch of salt

Instructions:

1. Heat a saucepan over a medium low flame and add in all the ingredients required to prepare the ice cream, except the sunflower seed butter.

2. Mix constantly until the cocoa is completely incorporated and it has a smooth consistency.

3. Take the saucepan off the heat and cool for a while before placing the saucepan in the freezer to cool completely. Should take about an hour.

4. Pour the contents of the saucepan into an ice cream maker and follow the instructions of the manufacturer.

5. When the ice cream is almost done, pour in the sunflower butter and allow it to get incorporated.

6. While the ice cream churns, place all the ingredients required to prepare the chocolate shell in a microwave proof bowl and heat on the low setting for about 30 seconds. Mix well to combine.

7. When the ice cream is ready, scoop into a bowl and spoon the chocolate shell mixture onto the ice cream scoop. Top with some sunflower butter if required.

8. Serve immediately.

9. Enjoy!

Sweet & Salty Fudge Bombs

Ingredients:

- ½ cup whole walnuts or pecans
- 2/3 cups pitted dates, about 8 dates
- ½ teaspoon vanilla extract
- 2 tablespoons Cocoa Powder
- For garnish: coarse sea salt, unsweetened shredded coconut

Instructions:

1. Place the dates, nuts, cocoa powder and vanilla extract in the jar of a food processor.
2. Pulse on high speed until it forms a paste.
3. Pour into a lined tin and refrigerate overnight.
4. Once the fudge is firm enough, cut into bite sized pieces.
5. Serve topped with a pinch of coarse sea salt or some shaved coconut.
6. Enjoy!

Mexican Chocolate Coffee Cake

Ingredients:

- 3 eggs
- ¼ cup extra virgin coconut oil, melted
- 3 tablespoons + ½ tablespoon coconut flour
- 3 tablespoons cacao powder
- 1 ½ oz. unsweetened chocolate, melted
- ¼ cup blackstrap molasses
- ¼ cup honey
- 1 teaspoon vanilla extract
- ¼ teaspoon salt
- ¼ teaspoon baking soda
- ½ teaspoon ground cinnamon
- ¼ teaspoon cayenne pepper or to taste

Instructions:

1. Crank up your oven to 325 degrees F. Lightly grease a 5 x 9 inch loaf pan and line it with a parchment sheet or wax paper. Lightly grease again with a little coconut oil.

2. Sieve the cocoa, cinnamon, salt, coconut flour, cayenne, baking soda and salt together in a small bowl. Ensure that there are no lumps.

3. Place the eggs, molasses, honey and vanilla extract together in the jar of a blender and pulse until well combined. Pour in the melted chocolate and coconut oil and pulse for another minute.

4. Slowly add the dry ingredients into the food processor, and blitz until well combined.

5. Pour the prepared batter into the lined and greased loaf pan and pop into the preheated oven for 45 minutes to 1 hour or until a toothpick poked in the center of the cake comes out clean.

6. Remove the pan from the oven and cool the cake in the pan.

7. Once cooled, extract from the pan and carefully peel away the wax or parchment paper.

8. Serve topped with some fresh fruits.

9. Enjoy!

Dairy Free Dark Chocolate Mousse

Ingredients:

<u>For the Mousse:</u>

- 2 ounces 71% cacao dark chocolate
- 1 ½ ounces water
- Pinch salt
- 1 ice cube tray worth of ice

<u>For the Whipped Cream:</u>

- ¼ can coconut milk, chilled
- ¼ teaspoon almond or vanilla extract

<u>For the Garnish:</u>

- Coarse sea salt

Instructions:

1. Freeze a small bowl and the beater whipping extension in the freezer before you start.
2. Heat a medium sized saucepan over a medium low flame. As the pan heats, break the chocolate into chunks and place it in the pan. Pour in the water and add a pinch of salt to it.
3. Whisk lightly to combine. Once the sauce gets a glossy sheen, turn off the heat.

4. Extract the ice cubes from the tray and place in a large bowl. Pour in about half a cup of chilled water.

5. Pour the prepared hot chocolate into a small bowl and place this bowl in the large bowl with the ice.

6. Using a wire whisk or an electronic blender, blend the chocolate until it gets a light and fluffy texture. Once the mousse acquires your desired consistency, remove it from the ice bath and refrigerate.

7. Remove the bowl and whipping extension from the freezer. Pour the chilled coconut cream into the frozen bowl.

8. Pour in the extract and then beat the cream until it gets a whipped cream like consistency. It should take about 5 minutes of beating.

9. Spoon the mousse into a serving bowl or glass, top with a dollop of the prepared "whipped cream" and serve immediately, garnished with a pinch of coarse sea salt.

10. Enjoy!

No Bake Banana Split Cake

Ingredients:

<u>For the Crust:</u>

- 1 ½ cups almond flour
- 1 teaspoon cinnamon
- 3 tablespoons sweetener
- ½ cup butter, melted

<u>For the Filling:</u>

- 1 8oz package cream cheese
- ½ cup confectioner's sweetener
- ½ cup butter, melted

<u>For the Topping:</u>

- 1 pint strawberries, sliced
- ½ banana, chopped
- ½ tablespoon lemon juice
- ¾ teaspoons unflavored gelatin
- 1 ½ tablespoons water
- 1 cup heavy whipping cream
- ½ teaspoon vanilla extract
- 1 ½ tablespoons sweetener
- Nuts (optional)
- Chocolate Sauce (optional)

Instructions:

1. Combine the almond flour, cinnamon, sweetener and butter together in a bowl. Press the prepared crust into the bottom of 9 x 13 inch pan.

2. Combine the confectioner's sweetener and cream cheese together in a mixing bowl. Add in the melted butter and mix until it gets a smooth texture.

3. Spread the prepared cream cheese filling on top of the prepared crust and set aside.

4. Combine the banana and strawberries together in a mixing bowl. Add in the lemon juice and mix well.

5. Spread the strawberry and banana mixture over the cream cheese mixture.

6. Start beating the whipping cream on a medium speed until it starts thickening.

7. Soften the gelatin in the water. Add the gelatin and the vanilla extract into the whipping cream and continue beating.

8. Spoon the whipped cream onto the strawberry and banana mixture.

9. Freeze overnight or until set.

10. Top with some chopped nuts or chocolate sauce if you wish.

11. Serve immediately.

12. Enjoy!

Healthy Strawberry Frozen Yogurt

Instructions:

- 2 cups frozen strawberries
- 1 ½ tablespoons honey or agave nectar
- ¼ cup plain Greek yogurt
- ½ tablespoon fresh lemon juice
- Sprig of mint, for garnish

Instructions:

1. Place the frozen strawberries, Greek yogurt, honey (or agave nectar) and lemon juice together in the jar of a food processor.
2. Process the ingredients until they form a smooth and creamy paste.
3. Serve immediately topped with a sprig of mint. (Or pour into an airtight container and refrigerate for up to one month).
4. Enjoy!

Salted Caramel Custard

Ingredients:

For the custard:

- 1 egg
- 1 oz. cream cheese, softened
- ½ cup water
- ¾ tablespoon granulated sugar substitute
- ¾ teaspoon caramel extract

For the caramel sauce:

- 1 tablespoon salted butter
- 2 tablespoons granulated sugar substitute
- ¼ teaspoon caramel extract, or to taste

Instructions:

To make the custard:

1. Crank up your oven to 325 degrees F and allow the oven to preheat for a few minutes. Grease a 6 oz. ramekin with some butter or line it with some parchment paper.
2. Place the egg, cream cheese, water, granulated sugar substitute and caramel extract together in the jar of a blender. Blend until well combined.
3. Pour the prepared custard mix into the prepared ramekin.
4. Place the ramekin on a cookie sheet and pop into the preheated oven.

5. Pour some hot water into the cookie sheet, about halfway up to the ramekin.

6. Bake for about 30 to 45 minutes or until the custard is set.

7. Remove the ramekins from the oven and cool before refrigerating. Chill for a minimum of 6 hours before serving.

To make the sauce:

1. Place the butter, caramel flavoring and sweetener in a microwave safe bowl. Place the bowl in the microwave and heat for about 30 seconds or place the ingredients in a small saucepan and heat over a low flame.

2. Whisk well until well combined.

3. Pour the sauce over the chilled custard and serve immediately.

4. Enjoy!

Delicious, Quick & Easy Cereal Treats

Ingredients:

- 1/2 (10.5 ounce) package miniature marshmallows
- 2 tablespoons butter
- 2 1/2 cups crispy rice cereal

Instructions:

1. Spray a 9 x 13 inch pan with some cooking spray or grease with some butter.
2. Place the butter and marshmallows together in a large microwave safe bowl.
3. Heat the marshmallows and butter together on high setting for about 3 minutes, stopping every 30 seconds to stir.
4. Keep heating until the marshmallows and butter are well combined and have a smooth texture.
5. Remove the bowl from the microwave and add in the cereal treats.
6. Lightly butter the back and front of a shallow spoon.
7. Use it to transfer the prepared cereal and marshmallow mix into the greased pan. Smoothen it out using the back of the spoon.
8. Place the pan in the refrigerator and chill for about 2 hours or until set.
9. Cut into squares and serve immediately.
10. Enjoy!

(Make these cereal treats kid friendly by topping them with some candies!)

Delicious Low Carb Rosettes

Ingredients:

- 1 egg

- 1/2 cup sifted all-purpose flour

- 1 1/2 teaspoons white sugar

- 1/2 cup milk

- 1/8 teaspoon salt

- 1/2 teaspoon vanilla extract

- Vegetable oil for frying

- Sifted confectioners' sugar

Instructions:

1. Place the eggs salt and sugar together in a large mixing bowl. Beat well until frothy.
2. Add in the sifted all-purpose flour, milk and vanilla extract and mix well until it forms a smooth and lump free batter.
3. Pour the vegetable oil into a fryer (or into a deep vessel) and heat it to 375 degrees F.
4. When the oil is hot, dip a rosette iron into the hot oil and keep it submerged in it for about 2 minutes or until heated through.
5. Lightly tap the rosette iron against the sidewall of the fryer or the vessel to remove the excessive oil from it.

6. Dip the hot rosette iron into the prepared batter, leaving about ¼ inch from the top of the iron.

7. Dip the batter coated iron back into the hot oil. Leave the rosette in for about 30 seconds or until the rosette is golden brown.

8. Remove the rosette iron from the hot oil and lightly tip it to drain the excess oil.

9. Push the rosette from the iron using a fork onto a rack covered with paper towels.

10. Reheat the iron for another minute and repeat the process 14 more times to make 15 rosettes in all.

11. While the rosettes cool, lightly dust them with confectioner's sugar.

12. Serve them after they've cooled down and have become crispy.

13. Enjoy!

Mini Fruit Filled Cream Cheese Tart Shells

Ingredients:

- 1/4 cup butter, softened
- 1 1/2 ounces cream cheese, softened
- 1/2 cup all-purpose flour
- ¾ cup fresh fruit (pineapple, apple, pear, melon, cut into bite sized pieces) [optional]

Instructions:

1. Place the cream cheese and margarine together in a large mixing bowl. Blend well until smooth.
2. Add in the flour and continue blending until just combined.
3. Place the prepared mix into the fridge and chill for an hour or two.
4. Crank up your oven to 325 degrees F and allow the oven to preheat for a while.
5. Lightly grease 12 mini muffin tins (or 12 molds of your 24 or 48 muffin tray) with some butter.
6. Shape the chilled dough into 12 even sized, one-inch balls.
7. Press the flour balls into the bottom of the muffin tin to prepare a hollow shell.
8. (If you wish to prepare stuffing filled tarts, spoon in your filling before baking)

9. Pop the muffin tins or muffin tray into the preheated oven and bake for about 25 to 30 minutes or until the crust is lightly browned.

10. Fill the tart shells with a tablespoon of your favorite fresh fruit pieces and serve immediately.

11. Enjoy!

Popcorn Macaroons

Ingredients:

- 1/8 teaspoon cream of tartar
- 1 cup popped popcorn
- 1/4 teaspoon baking powder
- 1 1/2 egg whites
- 1/8 teaspoon salt
- 1 tablespoon artificial sweetener, granulated (Splenda or the likes)
- Powdered artificial sweetener, for dusting

Instructions:

1. Crank up your oven to about 350 degrees F and allow the oven to preheat for a while.
2. Lightly spray a cookie sheet with some cooking spray or line it with a parchment paper.
3. Place the popped popcorn in the jar of a food processor or a blender and blitz until the popcorn separates into tiny pieces.
4. Place the egg whites in a large mixing bowl and whip until the egg whites are light and frothy.
5. Add in the salt, baking powder and cream of tartar and continue whipping until the egg whites form stiff peaks.
6. Slowly add in the granulated artificial sweetener and mix by hand.

7. Add in the tiny popcorn pieces and fold using a wooden spoon.

8. Scoop out about a teaspoon of the mixture and drop onto the prepared cookie sheet. Repeat with the remaining batter, leaving about an inch of space between two macaroons.

9. Pop the cookie sheet into the preheated oven and bake for 10 to 15 minutes or until the edges start browning.

10. Cool the tray before lightly extracting the prepared cookies from the cookie sheet.

11. Serve immediately, lightly dusted with powdered artificial sweetener.

12. Enjoy!

Chapter 11: Low Carb Smoothie Recipes

Cinnamon Roll Smoothie

Ingredients:

- 1 cup almond milk
- ½ teaspoon cinnamon
- 2 tablespoons vanilla protein powder
- ¼ teaspoon vanilla extract
- 1 teaspoon flax meal
- 4 teaspoons sugar substitute
- 1 cup ice

Instructions:

1. Place the almond milk and flax meal together in the jar of the blender and blend until well combined.
2. Add in the cinnamon, vanilla protein powder, vanilla extract and sugar substitute and blend for about 30 seconds or until it thickens.
3. Lastly, add in the ice and give it a whirl. Adding the ice last ensures that the smoothie remains thick and doesn't get diluted.
4. Serve immediately.
5. Enjoy!

Minty Green Protein Shake

Ingredients:

- ¼ avocado
- ½ cup spinach, fresh
- ½ scoop whey protein powder
- ¼ cup almond milk, unsweetened
- 6 drops of liquid sugar substitute
- ¼ tsp. peppermint extract
- ½ cup ice
- Optional: cacao nibs

Instructions:

1. Place the avocado, protein powder, spinach and almond milk together in the jar of a blender. Blend until it gets a smooth consistency.
2. Pour in the liquid sugar substitute and peppermint extract and blend again. Taste and adjust the sweetener.
3. Lastly, add in the ice and give it a whirl. Adding the ice last ensures that the smoothie remains thick and doesn't get diluted.
4. Serve immediately, topped with a few cacao nibs if required.
5. Enjoy!

Delicious Blueberry & Spinach Smoothie

Ingredients:

- 1 scoop vanilla protein powder
- 1/2 cup plain and full fat Greek yogurt
- 1/3 cup unsweetened almond milk
- 1/4 cup frozen blueberries
- 1 cup loosely packed spinach
- 1/3 cup ice

Instructions:

1. Place the Greek yogurt and almond milk together in the jar of the blender. Blend until smooth.
2. Add in the vanilla protein powder and spinach. Blend again until smooth.
3. Drop in the blueberries and blend until combined.
4. Lastly, add in the ice and give it a whirl. Adding the ice last ensures that the smoothie remains thick and doesn't get diluted.
5. Serve immediately, topped with some fresh blueberries.
6. Enjoy!

Coconut Mocha Frappe

Ingredients:

- 1 cup unsweetened coconut milk
- 1 teaspoon instant coffee
- ½ teaspoon unsweetened cocoa powder
- 1 drop of coconut extract
- 1 teaspoon stevia, or to taste

Instructions:

1. Place the coconut milk, cocoa powder and coffee together in a large cup. Mix well until the coffee is well incorporated.
2. Add in the coconut extract and stevia and mix well.
3. Place the cup in a freezer safe bowl and freeze.
4. Every 2 hours, remove the cup from the freezer and scrape it using a fork. Repeat until completely frozen.
5. Remove the cup from the freezer and leave it on the kitchen counter until it is slightly softer.
6. Pour the frappe into your blender and blend until smooth.
7. Serve immediately.
8. Enjoy!

Purple Detox Smoothie

Ingredients:

- ½ cup non-dairy milk, such as almond milk or coconut milk or water, chilled
- ¼ cup red cabbage
- ½ ripe banana, frozen but slightly thawed
- ¼ cup blueberries, frozen but slightly thawed
- 1 medium kale leaf, chopped

Instructions:

1. Pour the non- dairy milk or water into the jar of a blender.
2. Add in the red cabbage, banana, blueberries and kale. Blend until it gets a smooth consistency.
3. If you feel that there are bits of solids left, strain the smoothie before serving.
4. Pour the smoothie into a serving glass and serve immediately topped with some blueberries.
5. Enjoy!

Blackberry Banana Bliss Smoothie

Ingredients:

- 1 cup frozen blackberries, slightly thawed
- 2 - 3 drops vanilla extract
- ½ cup milk of choice, preferably almond milk or coconut milk, chilled
- ½ small banana, frozen but slightly thawed
- Sweetener to taste

Instructions:

1. Place the banana and blueberries in the blender and blend until it forms a smooth paste.
2. Pour in the milk and the vanilla extract and blend again until smooth.
3. Taste and adjust the sweetness.
4. Serve immediately topped with some blueberries.
5. Enjoy!

Key Lime Pie Style Protein Shake

Ingredients:

- ½ - 1 cup water, this will depend upon the consistency you want your shake to be
- 1/2 cup fat free cottage cheese
- 1 tablespoon lime juice
- 1 scoop vanilla protein powder
- 5 - 10 ice cubes, this will depend upon the consistency you want your shake to be, use less ice for a thinner consistency
- ¼ to 1 teaspoon of sugar substitute
- A few leaves of spinach or a few drops of green food coloring to give it a nice green color!

Instructions:

1. Place the cottage cheese, limejuice and water together in the jar of a blender and blend until smooth.
2. Add in the vanilla protein powder and sugar substitute and blend again.
3. Add your spinach or food coloring to give your shake some color.
4. Lastly, add in the ice and give it a whirl. Adding the ice last ensures that the smoothie remains thick and doesn't get diluted.
5. Serve chilled garnished with a sprig of cilantro.
6. Enjoy!

Blueberry Oatmeal Smoothie

Ingredients:

- 1 cup almond milk or coconut milk
- ¼ teaspoon vanilla extract
- ¼ cup regular oats
- 1 teaspoon maple syrup
- 1 teaspoon ground flax
- ½ cup blueberries
- ½ cup Greek yogurt, coconut flavored or vanilla flavored
- Ice cubes
- Homemade granola for topping, optional

Instructions:

1. Pour the almond or coconut milk into a large bowl. Add the oats to the milk and let them soak for about 7 to 10 minutes.
2. Pour the milk soaked oats into the jar of a blender and add in the Greek yogurt and ground flax. Blend well to combine.
3. Pour in the vanilla extract and maple syrup. Blend until smooth.
4. Add in the blueberries and blend until smooth.
5. Lastly, add in the ice and give it a whirl. Adding the ice last ensures that the smoothie remains thick and doesn't get diluted.
6. Serve immediately garnished with the homemade granola bar.
7. Enjoy!

Delicious Berry, Orange, Banana & Yogurt Smoothie

Ingredients:

- 1 cup mixed berries, frozen and slightly thawed
- 1 orange, peel removed and segmented
- 1 frozen banana, thawed
- 6 oz. vanilla Greek yogurt
- Ice cubes

Instructions:

1. Place the banana, orange segments and berries together in the jar of a blender and blend to form a smooth paste.
2. Add the Greek yogurt to the jar and blend until well combined.
3. Lastly, add in the ice and give it a whirl. Adding the ice last ensures that the smoothie remains thick and doesn't get diluted.
4. Enjoy!

Banaberry, Oat, & Baby Spinach Smoothie

Ingredients:

- 1 cup unsweetened almond milk, divided
- 1/4 banana, peeled
- 1 cup raspberries
- 1/2 cup rolled oats (raw)
- 3 cups raw baby spinach

Instructions:

1. Freeze the banana overnight until frozen to the core.
2. Pour about ½ cup unsweetened almond milk over the rolled oats and soak overnight or until the oats absorb all the milk.
3. Just before you start preparing the smoothie, remove the banana from the freezer and thaw for about 30 minutes or until slightly softened.
4. Place the frozen and thawed banana, raspberries, milk soaked oats, baby spinach and the remaining unsweetened almond milk in the jar of blender.
5. Blitz until it gets a smooth, creamy consistency.
6. Serve chilled, topped with a few raspberries.
7. Enjoy!

The Veggie Surprise

Ingredients:

- 1/2 medium zucchini
- 1/2 stalk celery
- 1/2 medium tomato
- 1 tiny slice of raw red onion
- 1 sprig fresh dill or ½ teaspoon dried dill
- 1/2 clove garlic
- Sea salt, to taste
- Cayenne pepper, to taste (optional)
- Black pepper, to taste
- 2 cups water, vary according to desired consistency

Instructions:

1. Place the zucchini, celery, tomato, red onion, fresh dill and garlic together in the jar of a blender. Blend until it forms a smooth paste.
2. Slowly trickle in the water, about 2 tablespoons at a time, and blend until smooth.
3. Repeat until it gets the consistency of your choice.
4. Add in the sea salt, black pepper, dried dill and cayenne (if using) to it. Blend once again to ensure there are no spice clumps in it.
5. Serve chilled garnished with a sprig of fresh dill.
6. Enjoy!

Peppermint Protein Punch

Ingredients:

- 2 cups cashew milk
- 2 scoops chocolate whey protein powder
- ½ teaspoon peppermint extract
- ½ cup baby spinach leaves, torn into bite sized pieces
- Ice cubes, crushed

Instructions:

1. Place the cashew milk, chocolate whey protein powder, peppermint extract and torn baby spinach leaves together in the jar of blender. Blend until smooth.
2. Add the crushed ice to two tall glasses. Pour the prepared smoothie over the crushed ice.
3. Serve immediately.
4. Enjoy!

Delicious Strawberry and Sage Smoothie

Ingredients:

- 2 cups unsweetened coconut milk
- 10 strawberries, frozen
- 4 tablespoons heavy cream
- 4 fresh sage leaves, divided
- 2 tablespoons sugar free vanilla syrup

Instructions:

1. Place the 2 sage leaves, frozen strawberries and heavy cream together in the jar of a blender. Blend until it forms a smooth paste.
2. Pour in the unsweetened coconut milk and sugar free vanilla syrup. Blend again until smooth.
3. Pour the prepared smoothie into 2 glasses and serve immediately topped with a fresh sage leaf each.
4. Enjoy!

Raspberry Cheesecake Smoothie

Ingredients:

- 2 cups almond milk
- 1 cup raspberries
- 2 oz. cream cheese
- 2 tablespoons sugar free vanilla syrup

Instructions:

1. Place the raspberries and cream cheese together in the jar of a blender. Blend until well-combined and there are no large pieces of raspberries left.
2. Pour in the almond milk and the sugar free vanilla syrup. Blend again.
3. Pour the smoothie into two tall glasses and serve immediately topped with some fresh raspberries.
4. Enjoy!

Delicious Chocolate & Orange Smoothie

Ingredients:

- 2 cups cashew milk
- 2 scoops chocolate whey protein powder
- ¼ teaspoon orange extract
- ½ cup baby spinach, torn into bite sized pieces
- Ice cubes, crushed

Instructions:

1. Place the cashew milk, chocolate whey protein, orange extract and baby spinach into the jar of blender.
2. Blend until well combined and smooth.
3. Pour the crushed ice into two tall glasses and pour the prepared smoothie over the crushed ice,
4. Serve immediately, garnished with a piece of peel of an orange. (Optional)
5. Enjoy!

Delicious Low Carb Hazelnut Coffee

Ingredients:

- 2/3 cup heavy cram
- 2 – 4 tablespoons of sugar free hazelnut syrup
- Ice cubes, crushed

Instructions:

1. Place the heavy cream and the sugar free hazelnut syrup together in the jar of blender. Blend until well combined.
2. Add the crushed ice into two tall glasses. Pour the prepared smoothie over the crushed ice.
3. Serve topped with some whipped heavy cream. (Optional)
4. Enjoy!

Conclusion

I would like to thank you once again for purchasing this book. I hope this book proved to be an informative read.

By now you would have realized all the benefits that a low-carb diet has got to offer. By simply changing your diet, you will be able to not only shed those extra kilos but also lead a healthier life. A diet doesn't have to mean starving yourself or cutting down on foods that you lie or enjoy eating. A diet simply means eating more of those things that your body has been designed to eat. It is about eating those foods that work well with your metabolism and not against it. By simply eating the right food you will be able to shed those extra kilos that have been piling up.

A low-carb diet simply restricts the amount of carbohydrates that you are used to consuming and by doing so it shifts your body's metabolism of burning carbs to generate energy to burning stored fat for providing energy. If you combine this diet with exercising you will be able to see the results in no time.

The recipes and the diet plan that have been given in this book are really easy to follow. Follow the tips that are given, the mental tactics to motivate yourself will keep you going and with the information provided in this book you will definitely be able to commit the mistakes that you might have.

You will need to put in some effort, stay committed to the diet and show some patience. The results would prove to be a pleasant surprise. So, what are you waiting for? Get started and all the best!